Adriana Budelon de Macedo

Nutritional Approach to Diabetes Mellitus in Pregnancy

Adriana Budelon de Macedo

Nutritional Approach to Diabetes Mellitus in Pregnancy

A Literature Review

ScienciaScripts

Imprint
Any brand names and product names mentioned in this book are subject to trademark, brand or patent protection and are trademarks or registered trademarks of their respective holders. The use of brand names, product names, common names, trade names, product descriptions etc. even without a particular marking in this work is in no way to be construed to mean that such names may be regarded as unrestricted in respect of trademark and brand protection legislation and could thus be used by anyone.

Cover image: www.ingimage.com

This book is a translation from the original published under ISBN 978-613-9-67862-4.

Publisher:
Sciencia Scripts
is a trademark of
Dodo Books Indian Ocean Ltd. and OmniScriptum S.R.L publishing group

120 High Road, East Finchley, London, N2 9ED, United Kingdom
Str. Armeneasca 28/1, office 1, Chisinau MD-2012, Republic of Moldova, Europe
Printed at: see last page
ISBN: 978-620-8-18187-1

SUMMARY

SUMMARY

The definition of gestational diabetes diagnosed in pregnancy in women without a diagnosis of diabetes before pregnancy, with hyperglycemia detected in pregnancy and with blood glucose levels that meet the WHO standards for diabetes in the absence of pregnancy. The aim of this study was to review scientific articles on the relationship between diet and glycemic control in pregnant women with diabetes mellitus. The results of the articles showed that women with GDM need to be monitored by a multi-professional team. It is important for pregnant women to undergo nutritional therapy even in the postpartum period in order to maintain their blood glucose levels.

Keywords: Gestational diabetes; nutritional treatment; treatment.

1 INTRODUCTION

According to the Ministry of Health (2006) Diabetes Mellitus (DM) is a group of metabolic diseases characterized by hyperglycemia and other complications, which may result from defects in the secretion or action of insulin.

The concept of Gestational Diabetes Mellitus (GDM) is hyperglycemia detected for the first time during the gestational-puerperal period, with blood glucose levels that do not meet the diagnostic standards for Diabetes Mellitus (WHO, 2013).

The American Diabetes Association (2016) currently defines GDM diagnosed in pregnancy as women without a diagnosis of DM before pregnancy, with hyperglycemia detected in pregnancy and with blood glucose levels that meet the WHO standards for DM in the absence of pregnancy.

Pregnancy hormones such as placental lactogen, progesterone, oestradiol, growth hormone and prolactin have an anti-insulin and counter-regulatory effect and can cause insulin resistance and diabetes in healthy pregnant women (LACROIX; KINA; HIVERT, 2013).

According to the International Association of the Diabetes and Pregnancy Study Groups (IADPSG) (2010) there are two different clinical situations: the diagnosis of DM in pregnancy, called Overt Diabetes, and GDM itself. It is also important to differentiate between GDM and women who become pregnant with previous DM.

GDM is associated with fetal macrosomia, prenatal complications, metabolic syndrome, type 2 DM and obesity in the adult life of the conceptus (SHEFFIELD et al. 2002; REECE EA, 2002).

According to the Brazilian Diabetes Society (2015), it is important for pregnant women diagnosed with GDM to receive nutritional therapy to control their blood glucose during pregnancy and in the puerperium, in order to avoid complications for the pregnant woman and her unborn child.

This research aims to review scientific articles on the relationship between diet and glycemic control in pregnant women with Diabetes Mellitus.

Diabetes mellitus is a common physiological alteration during pregnancy, affecting between 3 and 25% of pregnancies. The initial treatment for GDM is dietary advice and adjustments to the pregnant woman's diet. This helps to maintain adequate weight gain during pregnancy and keep blood glucose under control, as well as avoiding fetal macrosomia and other complications associated with GDM for the pregnant woman and the unborn child.

2. METHODOLOGY

This article is a Systematic Literature Review. The articles were searched using the following databases: Google Scholar, WHO, SCIELO, NCBI, SBD Archives, PUBMED, CAPES Journals and LILACS.

The index terms were: "null gestational DM"," diet gestational diabetes", "resistance insulin pregnancy", "risk to fetus of gestational diabetes", "dietotherapy diabetic pregnancy", "nutritional therapy of gestational diabetes mellitus", "diet in glycemic control in pregnant women with Diabetes Mellitus", "diet pregnancy diabetes", "nutritional management gestational diabetes", "gestational diabetes", "gestational diabetes carbohydrate counting" , low carbohydrate diet and Gestational "Diabetes Mellitus Treated with Diet, Metformin or Insulin".

The search revealed a total of (36,293) articles. Of these, a total of 91 articles were used as references in the review.

In Google Scholar, using the term "diet pregnancy diabetes", a total of (24800) results were found. Using the index term "gestational diabetes mellitus", (287) results were found, totaling (25087) results. Of these, (25000) articles were discarded in (phase 1) because they did not meet the selection criteria after reading the title and abstracts. Of these, 413 articles were selected for (phase 2) and of these, 15 articles were selected after reading.

In the Pubmed database, using the index term "low carbohydrate diet" (4550) results were found and using the term "gestational diabetes diet" (173) articles totaling (4723). Of these (4520) were discarded in (phase 1) after reading the title and abstract because they did not meet the selection criteria for the article. They went on to (phase 2) (203) articles which were translated and read and finally (14) articles were selected for the review.

In the NCBI database, a total of (6003) articles were found, and in (phase 1) (5050) articles were discarded. Then (953) articles were sent to (phase 2) and (43) articles were selected for the review.

In the Capes Journal (86) articles in total were excluded in (phase 1) (63) articles because the title and abstract did not meet the selection criteria for the review. (Phase 2) (23) articles were read and (3) articles were selected for the review.

The LILACS database found (11) results for the index term "nutritional therapy for gestational diabetes mellitus". (6) articles were discarded in (phase 1) because they did not meet the criteria for the review. There were (5) articles in phase 2, of which only (1) was used in the review.

The Scielo database found (15) results for the index "gestational diabetes", of which (12) were discarded after reading the title and abstract. They were then forwarded to (phase 2) (3) articles, of which (3) were selected.

In the (SBD) Archives, (454) results were found using the index "gestational diabetes", of which (450) were excluded in (phase 1), of which (4) went on to (phase 2), and these (4) articles were used in the review.

We used (12) articles from the World Health Organization.

3. RESULTS

3.1 DIABETES MELLITUS IN PREGNANCY

Diabetes Mellitus is a chronic metabolic disease that causes hyperglycemia. During pregnancy, it is responsible for complications such as fetal macrosomia (Figure 1) and fetal malformations. GDM is diagnosed during pregnancy. Pre-gestational DM is when the woman is already pregnant with type 1, type 2 or other DM (MINISTÉRIO DA SAÙDE, 2012).

GDM has long-term implications for the subsequent development of type 2 diabetes in pregnant women and an increased risk of obesity and glucose intolerance in the unborn child (BARBOUR et al. 2007).

According to Golbert and Campos (2008) the risk factors for GDM are: age over 25, obesity or excessive pregnancy gain, excessive central fat deposition, family history of DM, women with short stature < 1.5 m, and also who have had babies with excessive fetal growth or fetal macrosomia (**Figure 2**), hypertension or preeclampsia, fetal death and previous gestational DM.

Figure 1: Macrosomic baby weighing 5.475 kg due to GDM.

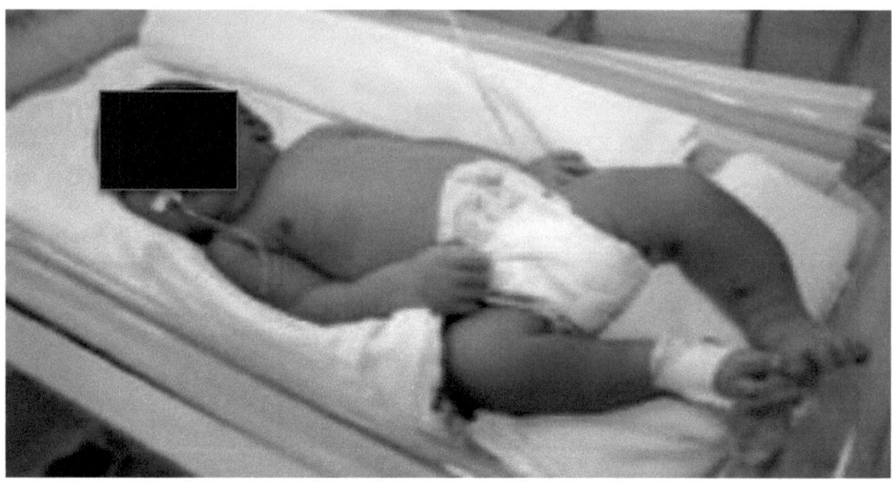

Source: http://www.infonet.com.br/noticias/saude/ler.asp?id=117324.

Figure 2: Newborn baby weighing 8 kg due to GDM.

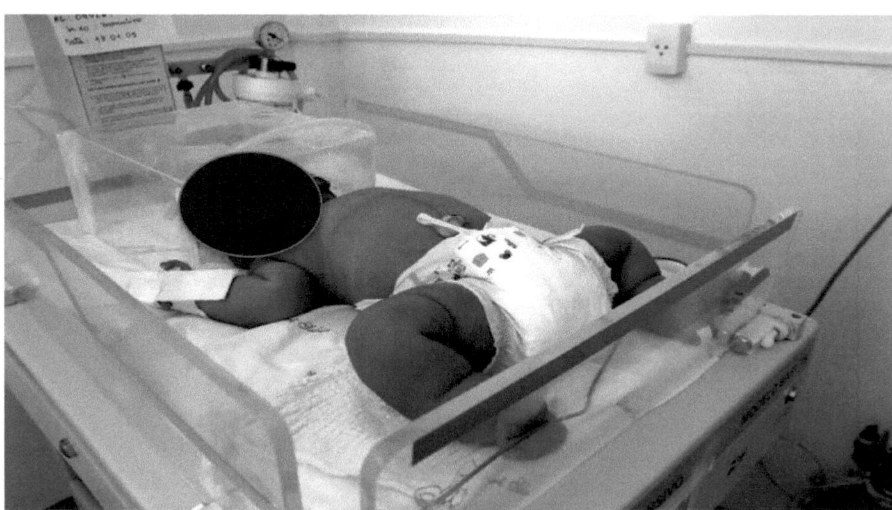

Source: https://www.megacurioso.com.br/recordes/39101-conheca-alguns-dos-maiores-bebes- who-were-born-in-the-world.htm.

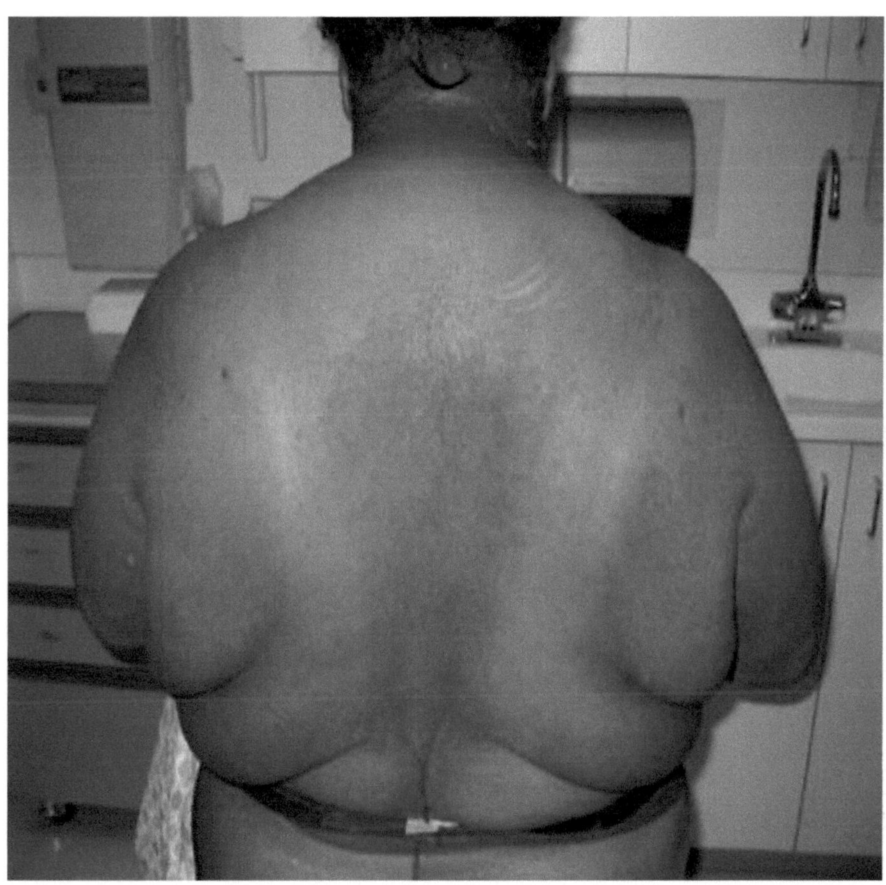

Source: https://bestpractice.bmj.com/topics/pt-br/424

The following are also considered risk factors for GDM: HbA1c $\geq$ 5.7% performed by ion exchange liquid chromatography (HPLC method), use of hyperglycemic drugs, Polycystic Ovary Syndrome, hypertriglyceridemia, Acanthosis Nigricans (**Figure 3**), Atherosclerotic Cardiovascular Disease (ADA, 2016).

3.2 Statistics

According to FEBRASGO (2018), the prevalence of GDM in the Unified Health System is approximately 18%. The International Diabetes Federation (IDF) calculates that one in six births

(16.8%) are to women with some form of dysglycemia in pregnancy, while 16% of these cases may be due to diabetes in pregnancy.

3.3   Diagnosis

The Brazilian Diabetes Society's Guidelines (2017-2018) state that screening for GDM is carried out in the first trimester of pregnancy at the first prenatal visit. It is also necessary to investigate DM beforehand. If a pregnant woman is diagnosed with GDM in the first trimester of pregnancy, this is considered to be pre-existing GDM (DM criteria for non-pregnant women).

Chart 1- Screening and diagnosis for GDM:

Fasting blood sugar	Blood glucose 2 hours after 75 g glucose overload	HbAlc	Random blood glucose
≥126 mg/dl	≥200mg/dl	≥ 6,5%	≥ 200mg/dl In the presence of symptoms.

Source: WHO; IADPSG.

Every woman with fasting glucose < 92 mg/dL is initially diagnosed with GDM. The protocol is to perform the oral overload test with 75 g of anhydrous glucose between 24 and 28 weeks of pregnancy, which diagnoses GDM. When at least one of the following values is altered (SBD, 2018):

Chart 2- Screening and diagnosis for GDM:

Fasting blood sugar	Blood glucose 1 hour after overload	Blood glucose 2 hours after overload
≥ 92 mg/dL;	≥ 180 mg/dL;	≥ 153 mg/dL.

Source: WHO; IADPSG.

Chart 3- Screening and diagnosis for GDM:

-	WHO (2013) Two altered values confirm the diagnosis.	National Institutes of Health (NIH) 2012. An altered value already confirms the diagnosis.	IADPSG (2010); ADA and SBD (2011); SBD, PAHO, FEBRASGO and MS (2017) Two altered values confirm the diagnosis.
Fasting	92 to 125 mg/dL	95 mg/dL	92 mg/dL
1 hour with 75 g of glucose.	180 mg/dL	180 mg/dL	180 mg/dL
2 hours with 75 g of glucose.	153 to 199mg/dL	155 mg/dL	153 mg/dl

Source: WHO: World Health Organization; NIH: National Institutes of Health; IADPSG: International Association of the Diabetes and Pregnancy Study Groups; ADA: American Diabetes Association; SBD: Brazilian Diabetes Society; PAHO: Pan American Health Organization; FEBRASGO: Brazilian Federation of Gynecology and Obstetrics Associations; MS: Ministry of Health.

Remember that the professional qualified to diagnose GDM is the doctor, not the nutritionist.

3.4 Pathophysiology

In the 1st trimester of pregnancy, insulin secretion increases, while insulin sensitivity remains unchanged, decreases or may even increase. However, in the 3rd trimester of pregnancy, maternal adipose tissue deposits decrease, while postprandial free fatty acid levels increase and insulin-mediated glucose disposal falls by 40% to 60% compared to the pre-pregnancy period. Chronic insulin resistance is a central component of the pathophysiology of GDM (CATALANO et al. 1993).

In pregnancy, postprandial hyperglycemia is a normal physiological condition. An increase in lipids in the bloodstream is also common: phospholipids, cholesterol, triglycerides and free fatty acids. These changes are part of a metabolic adaptation to provide energy for the fetus through lipolysis and also to prepare the pregnant woman's body for childbirth and lactation (O'SULLIVAN, 1982).

All these changes in the metabolism of hepatic glucose and lipids are due to the fact that the fetus is unable to make gluconeogenesis (synthesize glucose) in order to grow and depends on maternal nutrients via the placenta. It is through the placenta that glucose, glycerol and lipids reach the fetus and allow it to develop. Insulin resistance reduces glucose utilization, which in turn is redirected to the fetus. The pregnant woman's post-prandial hyperglycemia is also used to bring nutrients to the fetus (NEGRATO; GOMES; ZAJDENVERG, 2010).

Frenkel (1980) described this change in the metabolic pathway of glucose from the pregnant woman to fetal growth as: facilitated anabolism and accelerated catabolism. When GDM occurs, this excess of glucose and lipids for the fetus causes fetal hyperinsulinemia, which leads to macrosomia.

Insulin resistance may already be present before pregnancy in women with a history of GDM, but it increases even more during pregnancy. Insulin secretion is insufficient as a physiological mechanism to compensate for insulin resistance, leading to the hyperglycemia that is detected in pregnancy during prenatal care (CATALANO et al. 2002).

4. TREATMENT

4.1   Pre-pregnancy guidance

According to Kitzmiller et al. (2008) it is important for women who *already* have diabetes to plan their pregnancy beforehand. In order to plan their diet, carbohydrate counting, blood glucose monitoring and insulin therapy. Care should be taken to keep the glycated hemoglobin within normal limits for diabetic women. Pregnancy should only take place when the glycated hemoglobin is < 6%. Diabetics with a glycated hemoglobin >10% should be discouraged from becoming pregnant

According to Wahabi et al, (2012) pre-pregnancy care is important because it prevents congenital malformations and perinatal mortality in women with type 1 DM or GDM.

4.2 Nutritional treatment

Nutritional treatment is the first treatment measure for GDM (ADA, 2000).

In order to carry out the anthropometric assessment of the pregnant woman, the pre-pregnancy BMI classification must be carried out. Weight gain according to the pre-pregnancy BMI classification **(Table 4)** (IOM, 1994).

Chart 4: Pre-gestational BMI classification and weight gain for pregnant women.

Nutritional status	Weekly weight gain in the 1st trimester	Weight gain in the 2nd and 3rd trimester total	Total weight gain
Low weight	2.3 kg	0.5 kg	18kg
Suitable	1.6kg	0.4kg	16kg
Overweight	0.9 kg	0.3 kg	11.5 kg
Obesity	-	0.3kg	7.0 kg

Source: Institute of Medicine, (1992).

The Atalah curve is used to classify the nutritional status of pregnant women (ATALAH, 1997).

Franz et al. (1994) recommend that the weight gain of pregnant women with GDM should be 300 to 400 g per week from the second trimester onwards. The distribution of macronutrients should be: 55 g of carbohydrates, 15 to 20% of proteins and 30 to 40% of lipids.

According to the ADA, (2004) the distribution of macronutrients is 40 to 45% carbohydrates, 15 to 20% protein (at least 1.1 g/kg/day) and 30 to 40% lipids. It is also important to distribute the macronutrients over 6 meals/day in the diet throughout the day to avoid glucose spikes and hypoglycemia or ketosis. Generally, there are 3 main meals interspersed with 3 healthy snacks.

According to the ADA, (2018) there is no specific amount of macronutrients for women with GDM, it is recommended to use recommendations for pregnant women from the Dietary Reference Intakes (DRI), at least 175 g of carbohydrates, 71 g of protein and 28 grams of fiber. Vitamins and minerals are also in accordance with the DRIs for pregnant women.

The Brazilian Diabetes Society (2018) recommends in its latest guidelines that the calorie intake for pregnant women with GDM should be distributed as follows: 15% to 20% protein, 40% to 45% carbohydrates and 30% to 40% lipids. It is also important to divide this into 6 meals/day as follows: breakfast (10%), morning snack (10%), lunch (30%), afternoon snack (10%), dinner (30%), supper (10%).

According to Franz et al. (2002) in their article, bread and pasta have an effect on the overall glycemic index when compared to other foods. The authors recommend the intake of fiber, whole foods, fruits and vegetables for people with DM. They also emphasize that the amount of total carbohydrates in the diet is more important than the source and type of carbohydrate. Diet control in GDM is to achieve the maternal glycemic goal with an adequate nutritional outcome, with the pregnancy lasting 39 to 41 weeks and the baby being born weighing between 3 and 4 kg. The authors also state that an evening snack is necessary to prevent ketosis during the night and that glucose must always be monitored.

Table 5: Sweeteners allowed during pregnancy:

Sweetener	Safe quantity
Sucralose	15 mg/kg of weight
Saccharin	2.5 mg/kg of body weight;
Stevioside	5.5 mg/kg of weight;
Cyclamate	11 mg/kg of weight;
Aspartame	40 mg/kg of weight;
Acesulfame-K	15 mg/kg of weight;

Source: ADA, (2004).

In his study, Demétrio (2010) developed the Food Pyramid for eutrophic pregnant women **(Figure 1)** aged between 19 and 30, with portions recommended by the Food Guide for the Brazilian Population (2006) and Philippi et al (1996). To develop the pyramid, the author used two diet plans: one of 2,188 kcal for the 1st gestational trimester and another of 2,502 kcal for the 2nd and 3rd gestational trimesters. For overweight and obese pregnant women, the use of this food pyramid is not recommended, as well as the type of carbohydrate consumed and the presence of fiber in the diet of diabetic pregnant women needs to be considered.

Figure 4- Food pyramid for eutrophic pregnant women aged 19 to 30.

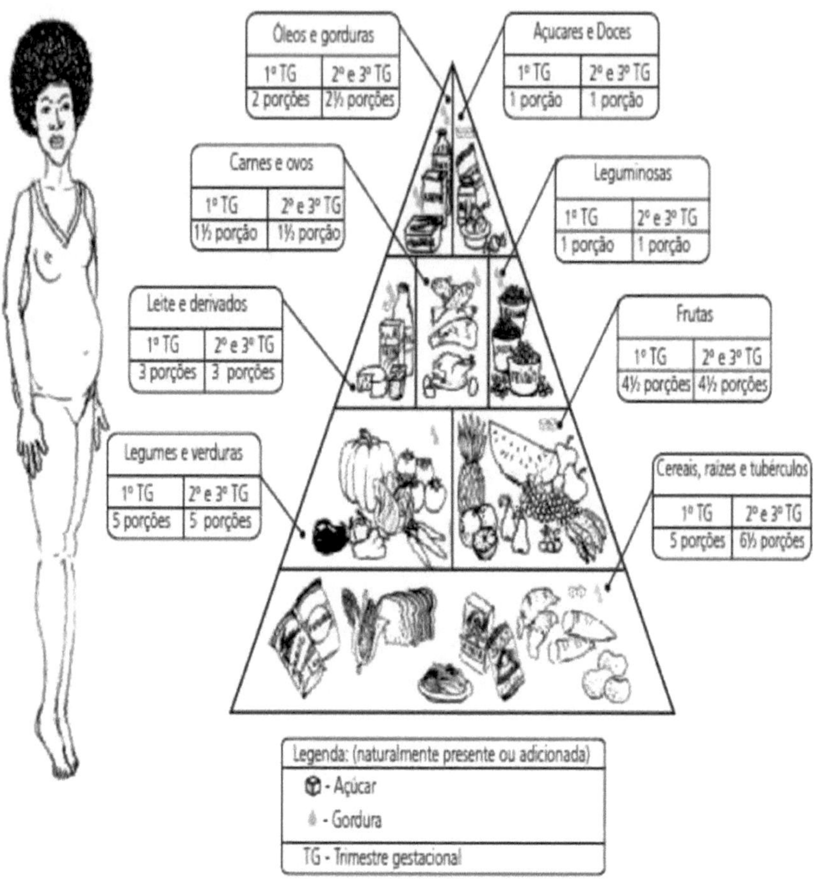

Figure 1. Food pyramid adapted for euthyroid pregnant women aged 19 to 30.

Source: Demetrio F.₁

Illustration: Fernando Souza.

Computer graphics finalization: Wesley Santos.

Portion data: Annex C of the food gu | a for the Brazilian population.

Source: Demétrio, F (2010).

According to Pereira and Reis (2013), micronutrients (calcium, magnesium, selenium, zinc and vitamin D) also interfere with insulin resistance, as they act on glucose homeostasis.

According to the Carbohydrate Counting Manual for Health Professionals (2009), the diet plan for pregnant women with GDM should be individualized, and carbohydrate counting can be carried out. The nutritionist needs to be aware of changes in the bolus/carbohydrate ratio throughout the day for patients on insulin. Calories are calculated according to BMI and classified according to the chart for pregnant women. Physical activity should also be encouraged.

4.2 Drug treatment

According to the "Gestational Diabetes" Consensus: Update (2017), drug therapy is indicated when glycemic control, has not been achieved with diet alone. The drugs used are: metformin, insulin and glibenclamide. It is the medical professional who decides on drug therapy.

Metformin is already used in Brazil as an initial treatment for GDM when glycemic control is not achieved through diet and exercise (WEINERT et al, 2011).

For Jovanovic et al. (2017) insulin therapy is indicated when nutritional treatment and physical exercise do not achieve glycemic goals.

In the study by Marques et al. (2014), 186 pregnant women with GDM found that there were no significant differences between the group that used metformin and the group that received diet treatment. In comparison with the rates of miscarriage, macrosomia, pre-eclampsia and congenital malformations. Of these patients, 32 used metformin, 121 used diet alone and 33 used insulin. Of the 32 patients who used metformin, 10 also had to receive insulin.

4.3 Puerperium monitoring

In the puerperium (postpartum) it is recommended to monitor blood glucose levels and basal insulin should be discontinued. Maintain the diabetes diet. Generally, women who have had GDM tend to normalize their glucose levels in the first few days after giving birth (PETTIT et al, 1997).

According to the Ministry of Health (2017), women with GDM have an increased chance of developing type 2 diabetes mellitus and glucose intolerance after childbirth.

Women who have had previous GDM have an increased chance of developing GDM in the current pregnancy, as well as developing type 2 DM. The risk factors for this are: fasting blood glucose in pregnancy above 100 mg/dl, non-white ethnicity, family history of type 2 diabetes, excessive weight gain during or after pregnancy, obesity, abdominal obesity, high-fat diet, sedentary lifestyle, and the use of insulin during pregnancy (DAMM et al, 1992).

If the puerperal woman develops hyperglycemia, the treatment indicated is insulin. Low-calorie diets should not be prescribed during the breastfeeding period (PRIDJIIAN and BENJAMIN, 2010).

The Oral Glucose Tolerance Test and fasting glucose should be done within six weeks of giving birth (WHO, 1999). In addition, a balanced diet and physical activity should be maintained (ADA, 2004).

According to Voormolen DN et al. (2018) it is important to screen newborns for hypoglycemia within the first 12 hours of life. For children of pregnant women with GDM. Because the incidence of hypoglycemia in neonates is recurrent both for pregnancies with diet-controlled DM and for pregnant women with DM1. Encouraging breastfeeding in the first hours after birth and the prevalence of breastfeeding for more than 3 months is also important for preventing the development of type 2 DM (ZIEGLER, 2012).

5. DISCUSSION

Table 1 and Table 2 show the articles from the Literature Review, organized in chronological order from 2011 to 2018.

Table 1: scientific articles presenting studies on the relationship between diet and control

glycemic levels in pregnant women with Diabetes Mellitus in terms of the type of study, the place where it was carried

out and the journal in which it was published, from 2011 to 2018.

Study	Year	Type of Study Location	Magazine
Nogueira et al.	2011	Hospital das Clinicas de Minas Gerais.	Revista de Medicina de Minas Gerais.
Karamanos et al.	2014	Observational study in 10 Mediterranean cities.	European Journal of Clinical Nutrition.
Teixeira et al.	2016	Case report from the maternity ward of the Hospital Universitario de Maceió .	GEP NEWS, Maceió.
Simeonova-Krstevska et al.	2018	Prospective randomized study conducted at the Department of Endocrinology and University Clinic of Obstetrics and Gynecology in Skopje.	Open Access Maced J Med Sci.
Kijmanawat A et al.	2018	Double-blind randomized controlled trial Thailand.	J Diabetes Investig.
Looman et al.	2018	Australian Longitudinal Study	Br J Nutr.
Gründahl et al.	2018	Retrospective study	J. Perinat. Med

Source: Estàcio de Sa University, 2018.

Table 2: scientific articles presenting studies on the relationship between diet and glycemic control in pregnant women with Diabetes Mellitus from "2011 to 2018".

Author	Year	Objectives	Study population	Period	Results	Conclusion
Nogueira et al.	2011	To assess the presence of risk factors, type and response to treatment, incidence of maternal, fetal and perinatal complications, and persistence of postpartum diabetes.	66 pregnant women with GDM at the Hospital das Clinicas de Minas Gerais.	Jan 2007 to Dec 2008.	Metabolic control was not satisfactory. 31 pregnant women (47%).	The population studied had poor metabolic control, due to the low socioeconomic level of the pregnant women attended.
Karamanos et al.	2014	To explore a possible relationship between the incidence of GDM and the eating pattern of the Mediterranean diet (MD).	In 10 Mediterranean countries, 1,076 pregnant women underwent a 75 g glucose TTOG at 24 to 32 IG. Eating habits were assessed using a questionnaire.	-	The incidence of GDM was lower in individuals with DM.	Adherence to a Mediterranean dietary pattern is associated with a lower incidence of gestational diabetes.
Teixeira et al	2016	To present a proposal for an individualized nutritional intervention for pregnant women with DM2 assisted in the maternity ward of the University Hospital of Maceió.	A 22-year-old pregnant woman with a gestational age of 29 weeks and previous DM2.	November 05-21, 2016.	Pharmacological and nutritional treatments were implemented simultaneously, given the patient's severe metabolic dyscontrol.	Nutritional treatment combined with pharmacological treatment has positive results in controlling the patient's weight and glycemic values.
Simeonova-Krstevska et al	2018	Compare DMG results treated with metformin, insulin or	48 women with GDM treated with metformin, 101 with insulin,	-	The number of SGA neonates was lower in the group treated with Metformin. The number	Metformin in women with GDM can improve maternal

		diet.	and 200 women on a diet		of SGA neonates and neonatal hypoglycemia was higher in the group treated with insulin.	and neonatal outcomes compared to those treated with diet or insulin.
Looman et al.	2018	To examine the association between the quantity and quality of carbohydrates in the pre-pregnancy diet and the risk of developing gestational diabetes mellitus (GDM).	3607 women aged between 25 and 30 without diabetes.	-	During 12 years of follow-up (2003-2015), 285 cases of GDM (4 - 6%) were reported in 6263 pregnancies among 3607 participants.	Higher fiber intake could reduce the risk of GDM. It is especially important to consider the source of carbohydrates
Gründahl et al.	2018	To compare the fetal brain structures evaluated in routine USG examinations during the 2nd and 3rd months of pregnant women with and without GDM.	231 pregnant women with GDM.	2001-2017 from a hospital in Germany.	The mean widths of the septum pellucidum and the lateral ventricles of the brain were greater in the fetuses of mothers with GDM.	GDM is associated with altered fetal brain development.

Source: Estàcio de Sa University, 2018.

The aim of this article was to present and discuss scientific papers on the relationship between diet and glycemic control in Gestational Diabetes Mellitus through original articles.

The articles were then read, selected and organized in ascending chronological order. Articles were selected from 2011 to 2018 in order to analyze how research has been carried out over these seven years on the subject of Nutritional Therapy for GDM. In the course of the article, the most important results of the selected articles are presented in relation to the theme of the Literature Review. Finally, we will conclude what the research currently shows about GDM in 2018.

In the study by Nogueira et al. (2011), 66 patients with a diagnosis of GDM were followed up at the Endocrinology and Metabology Service of the Hospital das Clinicas of the Federal University of Minas Gerais (UFMG). This study evaluated different forms of treatment for GDM: diet alone and insulin therapy alone. Metabolic control and the presence or absence of maternal-fetal complications, type of delivery and perinatal complications (28th week of pregnancy to the 7th day of life of the conceptus) were also assessed. The patients were given weekly guidance by the nutrition team, with diets of 30 kcal/kg ideal weight. Of the 66 pregnant women (35%) had varying degrees of pre-gestational obesity. After pregnancy (13%) had grade III obesity. In this study, metabolic control was unsatisfactory, with only 31 pregnant women (47%) being treated with diet alone. Insulin treatment was necessary in 36 patients (53%), of whom 7 used 1 dose of insulin, 11 used 2 doses and 17 used 3 doses or more of insulin a day. Of these 66 patients, 18% remained with diabetes postpartum. Due to the scarcity of resources in public health, primary care and delayed referral to referral centers.

For Ali et al. (2013) Nutritional therapy in GDM is the cornerstone of treatment for GDM. Carbohydrate is the main component that alters postprandial blood glucose levels, so the amount and type of carbohydrate are important, especially foods that are sources of fiber and low-glycemic index carbohydrates.

According to NICE (2015), the main treatment for GDM is diet therapy.

(2017) Nutritional therapy is the only treatment that will reach all women with GDM. Therefore, a diet based on complex carbohydrates with a low glycemic index, low in lipids and with an appropriate amount of protein in the diet, helps to maintain adequate blood glucose levels and to supply the nutrients necessary for a healthy pregnancy.

According to Kintiraki and Goulis (2018), early treatment of GDM reduces the risk of maternal and fetal complications. Treatment for GDM should be multi-professional and include lifestyle changes, physical activity, diet and, if necessary, drug treatment. Drug treatment is the secondary treatment for pregnant women who do not achieve glycemic control with diet and physical activity alone. The gold standard for drug treatment of GDM is insulin, combined with metformin and glibenclamide (an oral hypoglycemic drug), which are safe to use during pregnancy and in some countries are the first line of treatment for GDM. However, more long-term studies are still needed, especially for the health of the unborn child, and so it should only be used when the benefits outweigh the risks.

karamanos et al. (2014) conducted a study in hospital obstetric centers in 10 Mediterranean countries (Algeria, France, Greece, Italy, Lebanon, Malta, Morocco, Serbia, Syria and Tunisia). A total of 1076 pregnant women were studied and their eating habits were assessed using a questionnaire based on the Mediterranean food pyramid. The aim of the study was to assess the association between nutrient intake, individual intake and the pattern of food consumption of the Mediterranean diet and the development of GDM. In this study, it was observed that the group with GDM that had better adherence to the Mediterranean diet had better glucose tolerance. In hypothesis, the Mediterranean diet in pregnancy can improve glucose tolerance and reduce, to some extent, the incidence of GDM in pregnant women.

In the case study by Teixeira et al. (2016), the pregnant woman studied had DM2 prior to pregnancy. In this study, nutritional treatment was combined with pharmacological treatment and the result was an improvement in the patient's state of health.

In the study by Simeonova-Krstevska et al. (2018), the aim of the study was to compare the outcome of pregnancy (glycemic control, maternal and neonatal outcomes) in women with GDM who were followed up by the Outpatient Clinic of the University Clinic of Gynecology and Obstetrics in Skopje. A total of 349 pregnant women with GDM took part in the study, of whom 48 were treated with Metformin alone, (101) were treated with insulin and the rest were on a diet only. Blood glucose was self-monitored, the diet prescribed was for individualized DM and the calculation was 30 kg/kg/ ideal weight and overweight and obese pregnant women were calorie restricted to 25 kcal/kg/ ideal weight.

It was found that pregnant women treated with diet had a lower pre-gestational BMI, but greater gestational weight gain when compared to those treated with drugs or insulin. Mean glycosylated hemoglobin was lower in the Metformin-treated group and the diet-treated group than in the insulin-treated group. The study concluded that Metformin is effective in the treatment of GDM because the group treated with Metformin alone had lower weight gain and improved neonatal outcomes. However, it is not known whether the drug is completely safe for the fetus.

Looman et al. (2018) in their research on the type and source of carbohydrate ingested in the pre-pregnancy period, concluded that GDM can be prevented especially if women consume fiber during pregnancy.

In the study by Guillén et al. (2014) with twin pregnancies, it was concluded that GDM in twin pregnancies did not alter the weight of the newborn twins, but that GDM was associated with a higher risk of gestational hypertension and pre-eclampsia.

For Huet et al. (2018) obesity alone is a risk for maternal complications and is associated with GDM.

Berggren and Boggess (2013) state that treatment for GDM begins with diet and nutritional counseling. According to the authors, 50% of pregnant women with GDM can be treated with diet alone. The other half will probably need pharmacotherapy.

According to Weelden et al. (2018) the use of the oral hypoglycemic Metformin during pregnancy. It is associated with weight gain in the neonate. This is why more studies are needed on pre-natal exposure to Metformin.

Patti et al. (2018) state in their review that lifestyle changes (diet and physical activity) are important for the non-drug treatment of GDM. This is an excellent alternative. As for pharmacotherapy, when indicated, NPH insulin remains the best alternative. Oral hypoglycemic agents such as metformin and glibenclamide can be used during pregnancy, but are not yet well accepted by doctors.

In the research by Osinubi et al. (2018) with murines, the authors concluded that the oral hypoglycemic Glibenclamide is not safe to use in pregnancy to control gestational diabetes.

A retrospective analysis of (540) women with GDM who were medicated with the oral hypoglycemic Metformin in different trimesters of pregnancy. The study concluded that the use of Metformin in early pregnancy does not cause adverse effects on either the fetus or the pregnant woman (VANLALHRUAII et al. 2018).

In the non-randomized prospective interventional study on the possible harmful effects of Metformin during pregnancy. The study concluded that Metformin is safe to use during pregnancy. However, long-term studies with the conceptus should be carried out to verify possible harmful effects on the conceptus (SINGH et al. 2017).

In a systematic review of drug treatment for GDM, the authors concluded that the oral hypoglycemic agents Metformin and Glibenclamide are a good alternative when the patient does not accept insulin treatment or insulin administration is unfeasible. These drugs have been shown to be safe to use in pregnancy and lactation, but more studies are still needed on their safety in pregnancy (MAGON and Seshiah, 2011).

It is well known that the justification for the use of oral hypoglycemic agents in the treatment of GDM is based on scientific studies. When it comes to the administration of drugs in the gestational period, there is always the concern of teratogenicity due to the transfer of the drug to the placental barrier (LANGER, 2007).

According to Watson (2005), oral hypoglycemic agents are still not completely safe to use during pregnancy, and insulin should always be the choice.

The oral hypoglycemic Metformin is from the biguanide class and acts by decreasing glucose absorption and increasing peripheral utilization. Glibenclamide belongs to the sulphonylurea class and stimulates the release of insulin. Metformin is used in Polycystic Ovary Syndromes and is not teratogenic, i.e. it does not cause damage to the embryo (SILVA et al, 2009).

In a study of 404 pregnant women with GDM, the women were divided into two randomized groups, one group received insulin and the other group received Glibenclamide. This study found that Glibenclamide showed no change in the weight of the baby when compared to the insulin group. Glibenclamide was not found in umbilical cord serum. The study concluded that the oral hypoglycemic glibenclamide of the sulphonylurea class is a safe alternative for use in the treatment of GDM and can be used as an adjunct to insulin (LANGER et al, 2000).

In the research by Nguyen L; Chan; Teo, (2018) the authors state that Metformin crosses the placental barrier and can be found in umbilical cord blood. It reaches the same concentration as maternal plasma. Metformin is known to have pro-apoptotic effects, which is why more studies are needed on its use in early pregnancy.

For Dood et al. (2018) there is not enough scientific evidence for the use of Metformin in pregnancy. Dietary counseling and lifestyle guidelines are needed to improve maternal health.

For Su and Wang (2014) in their systematic review involving (1420) pregnant women with GDM, they found a higher prevalence of preterm birth in the group that used Metformin.

In the research by Moreno-Castilla et al. (2013) a randomized controlled open trial with a total of (152) women with GDM. The pregnant women were instructed to follow a low carbohydrate (40%) or (50%) carbohydrate diet. Food records were kept for 3 consecutive days. The following result was obtained: the control group that followed the low-carbohydrate diet did not reduce the need for insulin during pregnancy.

Bao et al. (2014) conducted a prospective study on pre-pregnancy dietary patterns. It concluded that women who ate a low-carbohydrate, high-protein, plant-based lipid diet had a lower incidence of GDM compared to women who ate a high-carbohydrate, animal-based fat diet.

A randomized study was carried out with pregnant women with GDM to investigate the influence of a low glycemic index diet on their postprandial glucose levels. They were given a low glycemic index diet for 5 days. They then obtained the following result: after the dietary intervention, the control group that received the low glycemic index diet had significantly reduced postprandial glucose values when compared to the other group that did not eat the diet (HU et al, 2014).

Another study was carried out at the Maternal Primary Care Center at Guangdong General Hospital in China with (95) pregnant women with GDM. In this study, they were divided into two groups: one control group received an individualized diabetes diet and the other group received a low glycemic index diet with intensive control of calorie intake, in order to assess whether a low glycemic index diet interferes with glycemic control and maternal blood lipid levels. The results were positive: the group that received the low glycemic index diet for two weeks had better control of blood glucose and blood lipids when compared to the other group that received the diabetes diet without controlling the glycemic index of the food (MA et al, 2015).

In a systematic review, Spaight et al. (2016) concluded that nutritional therapy for pregnant women with GDM and physical activity are the basis for the treatment of GDM. They help to reduce blood glucose levels and/or reduce insulin use. However, in some cases it is still necessary to use metformin and glibenclamide.

In the study by Maruichi et al. (2012) after the diagnosis of GDM, pregnant women should start nutritional therapy and physical activity, and if hyperglycemia is not controlled, insulin therapy should be started.

For Alfadhli (2015) the priority treatment for GDM is diet and physical exercise. If this isn't enough, insulin therapy and pharmacotherapy begin.

Kim's (2014) review shows that even after giving birth, women need to maintain healthy lifestyle habits, eat a balanced diet and exercise, even if their blood glucose levels return to normal.

A retrospective study was carried out in Japan on pregnant women with GDM. In this study, the women were divided into 3 groups according to their pre-gestational BMI. Of these women (426) were classified as overweight and (372) as obese. Women with GDM who were obese during pregnancy had large-for-gestational-age (LGA) newborns. The study suggests that medical and nutritional interventions in obese pregnant women with GDM help to reduce the incidence of SGA newborns (SUGIYAMA, 2014).

Krejci (2016) in his study concluded that diet and physical activity for pregnant women with low-risk GDM is an effective treatment to keep glucose levels under control and if pharmacotherapy is necessary, small doses are used. Early treatment with diet and physical activity reduces the risk of maternal and fetal complications.

The epidemic of obesity and DM2 in the world increases the risk of developing GDM, especially in underdeveloped countries such as Asia. Because GDM is a serious metabolic complication in pregnancy, it can cause fetal malformations and maternal complications. The authors of the systematic review on GDM emphasize the importance of campaigns to raise awareness among women about proper nutrition and a healthy lifestyle (JAWAD and EJAZ, 2016).

In the observational, descriptive and cross-sectional study by Souza et al. (2014) carried out with (11) pregnant women with GDM, the authors concluded that nutritional therapy is important for good glycemic control during pregnancy. And that prenatal nutritional status such as overweight/obesity and weight gain greater than recommended during pregnancy are factors that cause GDM and make it difficult to control blood glucose.

Gründahl et al. (2018) studied 231 fetuses of women with GDM between 20 and 41 weeks of gestation. Ultrasound showed that GDM can cause changes in the brain development of the fetus. In this study, the width of the pellucid septum and the lateral ventricles (LV) of the brain were greater in the fetuses of diabetic pregnant women (Figure 5). The size of the pellucid septum is 5.68 mm and the LV is 8.41 mm. The normal size is 3.29 mm for the pellucid septum and 5.39 mm for the VL. Of the 231 pregnant women in the study, 61 were treated only with diet and 82 with insulin.

Figure 5- Size of the septum pellucidum and lateral ventricle of the brain of a conceptus of a pregnant woman with GDM.

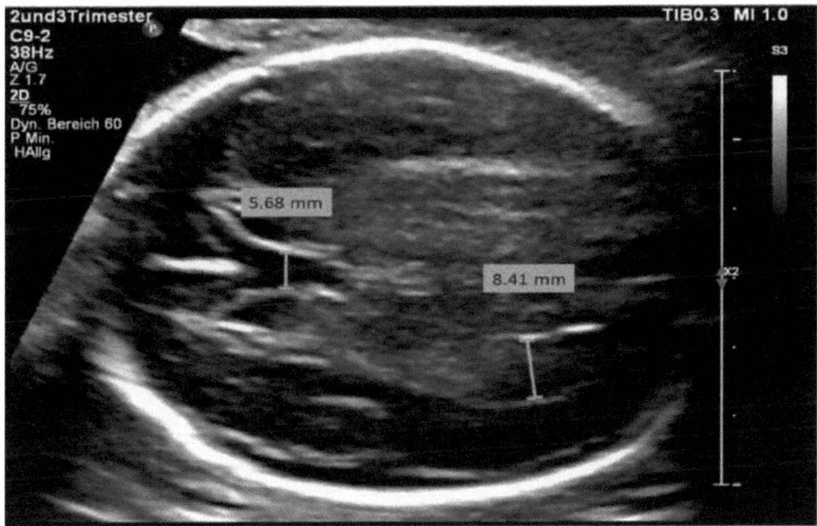

Source: Gründahl et al. (2018).

In the systematic review by Martis et al. (2018), the authors concluded that changes in lifestyle habits (diet and physical activity) were more effective in maintaining blood glucose levels, as well as preventing fetal macrosomia. Insulin therapy was associated with hypertensive disorders during pregnancy.

Few studies have looked at the relationship between pre-pregnancy diet and the development of gestational diabetes. In a cohort study carried out in Canada with (1545) women. The participants completed a food frequency questionnaire before pregnancy. This study found that nutritional intervention before pregnancy reduces the likelihood of maternal complications such as GDM and hypertension (JARMAN, 2018).

For Yang (2018), dietary factors are factors that can be modified. A varied diet based on legumes, vegetables and cereals helps maintain and gain adequate weight during pregnancy.

During labor, capillary blood glucose should be monitored every hour. If general anesthesia is administered, capillary blood glucose should be monitored every 30 minutes. After removal of the placenta, intravenous insulin should be reduced by at least 50%. An additional snack may be necessary after delivery, especially for breastfeeding. Capillary glucose should be monitored 1 hour before and 1 hour after the meal up to 24 hours after delivery. Women who had previous DM can continue taking Metformin after giving birth (DASHORA et al, 2018).

Yamashita et al. (2018) believe that pre-gestational BMI and pre-gestational fasting glucose levels could be used to screen pregnant women with GDM, who need intensive care during pregnancy, during prenatal care. And thus start taking care of their diet from the beginning of prenatal care.

6. FINAL CONSIDERATIONS

The results of the articles show that women with GDM need to be monitored by a multi-professional team. It is important for pregnant women to undergo nutritional therapy even in the postpartum period in order to maintain their blood glucose levels.

Based on the scientific articles studied, it can be concluded that diet and physical activity are essential for controlling GDM, as well as contributing to preventing women from developing DM in the postpartum period and to long-term cardiovascular health. Drug treatment is indicated when necessary and should be prescribed by the doctor.

And finally, to advise pregnant women on the importance of breastfeeding (BF) during pregnancy. As well as the importance of breastfeeding in the first few hours after giving birth.

7. REFERENCES

ALFADHLI EM. Gestational diabetes mellitus. **Saudi Med J**. v.36, n. 4, p. 399-406. 2015.

ALI, H; PAPAKONSTANTINOU, E; MESMOUDI, N. Diet and Carbohydrate Food Knowledge in Gestational Diabetes: Challenges and Opportunities for Lifestyle Interventions. **Nutrition and Diet in Maternal Diabetes**. p. 413-427. 2013.

AMERICAN DIABETES ASSOCIATION. Medical management of pregnancy complicated by diabetes. 3rd ed. **Clinical Education** Series. Arlington; 2000.

Management of Diabetes in Pregnancy: Standards of Medical Care in Diabetes. **Diabetes Care**. 41(1): S137-S143. Jan. 2018.

. Position of the American Dietetic Association: Use of Nutritive and Nonnutritive Sweeteners. **J Am Diet Assoc**. v. 104, n. 2, p.255-275, Feb.2004.

. Classification and Diagnosis of Diabetes. **Diabetes Care**. v. 39, n.1, p. 13-22 , 2016.

ATALAH SE, CASTILLO LC, CASTRO SR, ALDEA PA. Proposal for a new standard of nutritional assessment in pregnant women. **Rev Med.** Chile, 1997

BARBOUR, LA et al. Cellular mechanisms for insulin resistance in normal pregnancy and gestational diabetes. **Diabetes Care** 2:S112-9.Jul. 2007.

BRAZIL. Screening and diagnosis of gestational diabetes mellitus in Brazil.

Brasilia/ Ministry of Health, 2017; 36p. Available at:<

http://www.diabetes.org.br/profissionais/images/pdf/diabetes-gestacional-relatorio.pdf.> Accessed: Jun 2018.

. Caderno de Atençâo Bàsica: Diabetes Mellitus, 2006; 56 p. Available at: <http://bvsms.saude.gov.br/bvs/publicacoes/diabetes_mellitus.PDF>. Accessed on: Aug 2018.

. Prenatal and Puerperium: qualified and humanized care. Technical manual. Brasilia, 2006. Available at: <http://bvsms.saude.gov.br/bvs/publicacoes/manual_pre_natal_puerperio_3ed.pdf>.

Accessed on: Aug 2018.

Diretrizes da Sociedade Brasileira de Diabetes/Sociedade Brasileira de Diabetes, 204-2015; 390 p. Available at: https://www.diabetes.org.br/publico/images/2015/area-restrita/diretrizes-sbd-2015.pdf.

Accessed on: June 2018.

. Carbohydrate Counting Manual for People with Diabetes, 2016; 56p. Available at: <https://www.diabetes.org.br/publico/images/manual-de-contagem-de-   carboidrato2016.pdf>. Accessed on 03 Sep 2018.

BAO, W et al. Prepregnancy low-carbohydrate dietary pattern and risk of gestational diabetes mellitus: a prospective cohort study. **The American Journal of Clinical Nutrition.** v. 99, n. 6, p. 1378-84. Jun. 2014.

BERGGREN EK; BOGGESS KA. Oral agents for the management of gestational diabetes. **Clin obstet gynecology journal.** V. 56, n. 4, p. 827-36, Dec, 2013.

CATALANO, PM et al. Carbohydrate metabolism during pregnancy in control subjects and women with gestational diabetes. **Am J Physiol.** v. 64, n.1, p. 60- 70, Jan, 1993.

. Longitudinal changes in glucose metabolism during pregnancy in obese women with normal glucose tolerance and gestational diabetes mellitus. **Am J Obstet Gynecol.** v. 180, n. 4, p. 903-16, Apr, 1999.

. Downregulated IRS-1 and PPARγ in obese women with gestational diabetes: relationship to FFA during pregnancy. **Am J Physiol Endocrinol Metab**. v. 282, p. 522-523, Nov, 2001.

CENTERS FOR DISEASE CONTROL. Recommendations for use of folic acid to reduce the numbers of cases of spina bifida and other neural tube defects. MMWR **Recommendations and Reports.** v. 41, p. 1-7, 1992.

CLASSIFICATION AND DIAGNOSIS OF DIABETES. **Diabetes Care**. Suppl 1, v.

39. P. 13-22. 2016.

CONNEL FA, VADHEIM C, EMANUEL I. Diabetes in pregnancy: A population based study of incidence, referral for care and perinatal mortality. **Am J Obstet Gynecol**. N. 151p. 598-603.1985.

COUTO, A., et al. "Gestational diabetes" consensus: 2017 update. Portuguese Journal of Diabetes, Vol. 12, p.24-38, 2017

DAMM P, KUHL C, BERTELSEN A, MOLSTED-PEDERSEN L. Predictive factors for the development of diabetes in women with previous gestational diabetes mellitus. **Am J Obstet Gynecol**. v. 167, n. 3, p. 607-16, 1992.

DASHORA U et al. Managing hyperglycaemia during antenatal steroid administration, labor and birth in pregnant women with diabetes. **Diabetic Medicine**. V. 35, n. 8, p. 1005-1010. Aug. 2018.

DEMÉTRIO F. Food pyramid for eutrophic pregnant women aged 19 to 30. **Revista de Nutriçâo**, Campinas, v. 23, n. 5, 2010.

DOOD, JM et al. Metformin for women who are overweight or obese during pregnancy for improving maternal and infant outcomes. **Cochrane Database Syst**. Jul. 2018.

FEBRASGO. Brazilian Federation of Gynecology and Obstetrics Associations. Screening and Diagnosis of Diabetes Mellitus in Brazil. 2017. Available at: <https://www.diabetes.org.br/profissionais/images/pdf/diabetes-gestacional-relatorio.pdf>. Accessed on: Aug 2018.

FIGO. The_International

Federation_of_Gynecology_and_Obstetrics_FIGO_Initiative_on_gestational_diabetes_ mellitus_A_ pragmatic_guide_for_diagnosis_management_and_care. 2015. Available at: < www.researchgate.net/publication/282435651_>. Accessed on: 2 Aug. 2018.

FRANZ MJ, HORTON et al. Nutrition principles for the management of diabetes and related complications. **Diabetes Care.** v. 17, n. 5, p. 490-518, 1994.

FRANZ MJ et al. Evidence-Based Nutrition Principles and Recommendations for the Treatment and Prevention of Diabetes and Related Complications. **Diabetes Care.** v. 25, n. 1, p.148-198, Jan, 2002.

FRENKEIL, N. Banting Lecture 1980. Of pregnancy and progeny. **Diabetes.** v. 29, n.12, p.1023-35, Dec, 1980.

GOLBERT, Airton; CAMPOS, Maria Amélia A.. Type 1 diabetes mellitus and pregnancy. **Arq Bras Endocrinol Metab**, Sâo Paulo , v. 52, n. 2, p. 307314, Mar. 2008 .

GUILLEN MA et al. Influence of gestational diabetes mellitus on neonatal weight outcome in twin pregnancies. **Diabet Med**. Spain, v. 31, n. 12, p. 1651-6, Dec. 2014.

GRÜNDAHL , F Ruth et al. Fetal brain development in diabetic pregnancies and normal controls. **Journal neonatal perinatal med**, Germany, Jul. 2018.

HERNANDEZ, T et al. Higher Complex Carbohydrate Diets in Gestational Diabetes.

Nutrition and Diet in Maternal Diabetes. p. 429-450, 2017.

HU, ZG et al. A low glycemic index staple diet reduces postprandial glucose values in Asian women with gestational diabetes mellitus. **J Investig Med.** Dec. 2014.

HUET, Justin et al. Joint impact of gestational diabetes and obesity on perinatal outcomes. **Journal of Gynecology Obstetrics and Human Reproduction**. France. Aug, 2018.

HUI, AL et al. Barriers and coping strategies of women with gestational diabetes to follow dietary advice. **Woman Birth**. v. 27, n.4, p. 292-7, Dec, 2014.

INTERNATIONAL DIABETES FEDERATION. IDF Diabetes atlas. 6th ed. Brussels, Belgium: International Diabetes Federation. 2013. Available at:< https: //www.idf.org/e-library/epidemiology-research/diabetes-atlas/19-atlas-6th- edition.html>. Accessed on: Aug 2018.

IOM (Institute of Medicine) and NRC (National Research Council). Weight Gain During Pregnancy: Reexamining the Guidelines. Washington, DC: The National Academies Press; 2009.

IADPSG. Consensus Panel. International Association of Diabetes and Pregnancy Study Groups. Recommendations on the Diagnosis and Classification of Hyperglycemia in Pregnancy. **Diabetes Care**. V. 33, n. 3, p. 676-682. 2010.

JARMAN M et al. Dietary Patterns Prior to Pregnancy and Associations with Pregnancy Complications. **Nutrients**.v.10, n. 7, p. 914. Canada. 2018.

JOVANOVIC L, ILIC S, PETTITDJ et al. Metabolic and immunologic effects of insulin lispro in gestational diabetes. **Diabetes Care**. v. 22, n. 9, p. 1422-27, Sep, 1999.

KARAMANOS, B et al. Relation of the Mediterranean diet with the incidence of gestational diabetes. **Eur J Clin Nutr**. v. 68, n. 1, p. 8-13. Jan. 2014.

KIM, C. Maternal outcomes and follow-up after gestational diabetes mellitus. Kim C1.**Diabet Med.** V.31, n.3, p. 292-301. Mar. 2014.

KINTIRAKI, E; GOULIS, DG.. Gestational diabetes mellitus: Multi-disciplinary treatment approaches. **Metabolism**. 2018.

KITZMILLER JL et al. Managing preexisting diabetes for pregnancy: summary of evidence and consensus recommendations for care. **Diabetes Care**. v. 31. n. 5, p.106079. 2008.

Krejci H. Gestational Diabetes Mellitus. **Vnitr Lek.** 62(11) : S52-61. 2016.

LACROIX M , Kina E, Hivert MF. Maternal/Fetal Determinants of Insulin Resistance in Women During Pregnancy and in Offspring Over Life. **Curr Diab**. v. 13, n. 2, p.238244. Apr. 2013.

LANGER, O. Oral anti-hyperglycemic agents for the management of gestational diabetes mellitus. **Obstet Gynecol Clin North Am**. v.34, n. 2, p. 255-274. Jun. 2007.

LANGER O,et al. A comparison of glyburide and insulin in women with gestational diabetes mellitus. **N Engl J Med**. V. 343, n. 16, p. 1134-8.2000

LOOMAN, Moniek et al. Pre-pregnancy dietary carbohydrate quantity and quality, and risk of developing gestational diabetes: the Australian Longitudinal Study on Women's Health. **Br J Nutr**. p.1-10. Apr. 2018.

MA, W J et al. Intensive low-glycaemic-load dietary intervention for the management of glycaemia and serum lipids among women with gestational diabetes: a randomized control trial. **Public health nutr journal.**v.18, n. 8, p. 1506-13. Jun. 2015.

MACHADO, Raphaela Corrêa Monteiro et al. The symbolic dimension of prenatal nutrition care in diabetes Mellitus. **Rev. Nutr.**, Campinas, v. 30, n. 6, p. 703711, Dec. 2017.

MAGON, Navneet; SESHIAH , V. Gestational diabetes mellitus: Non-insulin management. **Indian J Endocrinol Metab.** v. 15, n.4, p. 284-293. 2011.

MARQUES P. CARVALHO MR, PINTO L E GUERRA S. Metformin Safety in the Management of Gestational Diabetes. **Endocr Pract**. v. 20, n. 10, p. 1022-31. 2014.

MARUICHI, Marcelo Damàsio et al. Gestational diabetes mellitus. **Arq Med Hosp Fac Cienc Med Santa Casa**. V. 57, n. 3, p. 124-8. 2012.

MARTIS Ruth et al. Treatments for women with gestational diabetes mellitus: an overview of Cochrane systematic reviews. **Cochrane library**. Aug, 2018.

MATHIESEN ER, HOD M, IVANISEVIC, M et al. Maternal efficacy and safety outcomes in a randomized controlled trial comparing insulin detemir with NPH insulin in 310 pregnant women with type 1 diabetes. **Diabetes Care**. v.35. n. 10, p. 2012-2017, Oct, 2012.

METZGER et al. Hyperglycemia and adverse pregnancy outcomes. **N Engl J Med**. Chicago. v.358, n. 19, p. 1991-2002. 2008.

METZGER BE, Gabbe, et al. International association of diabetes and pregnancy study groups recommendations on the diagnosis and classification of hyperglycemia in pregnancy. **Diabetes Care**. v.33, n. 3, p. 676-82. 2010.

MILLS J, KNOPP RH, SIMPSON JL ET AL. Lack of relation of increased malformations rates in infants of diabetic mothers to glycemic control during organogenesis. **N Engl J Med**. v. 318, p. 671-6. 1988.

MORENO-CASTILLA C et al. Low-carbohydrate diet for the treatment of gestational diabetes mellitus: a randomized controlled trial. **Diabetes Care**. v. 36, n. 8, p. 22338.2013.

National Academy of Sciences, Institute of Medicine, Food and Nutrition Board, Committee on Nutritional Status During Pregnancy and Lactation, Subcommittee for a Clinical Application Guide. Nutrition During Pregnancy and Lactation: An Implementation Guide. Washington, DC: National Academies Press; 1992.

National Institute for Health and Clinical Excellence. Diabetes in Pregnancy: Management of Diabetes and its Complications from Preconception to the Postnatal Period. NICE Guideline NG3. London (UK): National Institute for Health and Care Excellence, 2015.

NEGRATO C et al. Dysglycemias in pregnancy: from diagnosis to treatment. Brazilian consensus statement. **Diabetol Metab Syndr.** v. 27. n. 2. 2010.

NGUYEN L; CHAN SY; TEO AKK. Metformin from mother to unborn child - Are there unwarranted effects? **Ebiomedicine.** Singapore. Aug. 2018.

NOGUEIRA AI et al. Gestational diabetes: profile and evolution of a group of patients at the Hospital das Clinicas de UFMG. **Rev. Med. Minas Gerais,** Belo Horizonte, v. 21, n. 1,p. 32-41. 2011.

OSINUBI A. et al. A comparison of the anti-diabetic potential of d-ribose-l-cysteine with insulin, and oral hypoglycaemic agents on pregnant rats. **Toxicology Reports.** Nigeria. Aug. 2018.

PATTI et al. Pharmacotherapy for gestational diabetes. **Expert Opin Pharmacother**. Aug. 2018.

PEREIRA, KM; REIS, LBSM. Glycemic control during pregnancy and the interference of micronutrients: magnesium, selenium, zinc, calcium and vitamin D. **Com. Ciências Saùde**. v. 24,L n.2, P.169-178. 2013.

PETTITT DJ et al. Breastfeeding and incidence of non-insulin-dependent diabetes mellitus in Pima indians. The Lancet. n. 350, p. 166-8. 1997

PHILIPPI, Sonia Tucunduva et al . Adapted food pyramid: a guide to food choice. **Rev. Nutr.**, Campinas, v. 12, n. 1, p. 65-80, Apr. 1999.

PRIDJIIAN G, BENJAMIN TD. Update on Gestational Diabetes. **Obstet Gynecol Clin N AM.** v. 37, n. 2, p. 255-67. Jun. 2010

REECE EA et al. A consensus report of the Diabetes in Pregnancy Study Group of North America Conference, Little Rock, Arkansas, May 2002.

J Matern Fetal Neonatal Med., v. 12, n.6 . p. 362-4. Dec. 2002.

RAY JG, O'Brien TE, Chan WS. Preconception care and the risk of congenital anomalies in the offspring of women with diabetes mellitus: A meta-analysis. **QJM**. v. 94, n.8, p. 435-44. 2001.

O'SULLIVAN, MD. Body Weight and Subsequent Diabetes Mellitus. **Jama**. v. 248, n. 8, p. 949-952. Aug. 1982.

SHEFFIELD JS et al. Maternal diabetes mellitus and infant malformations. **Obstet Gynecol**. v. 100, n. 5, p. 925-30. Nov. 2002.

SCHMALFUSS, Joice Moreira; BONILHA, Ana Lucia de Lourenzi. Implications of diet restrictions in the daily lives of women with gestational Diabetes Mellitus / Implicações de las restricciones alimentares en la vida diaria de mujeres con Diabetes Mellitus en la gestación. **Revista Enfermagem UERJ**, Rio de Janeiro, v. 23, n. 1, p. 39-44, jan-feb. 2015.

SILVA, Jean Carl et al. Oral hypoglycemic agents in pregnancy: metformin versus glibenclamide. **Femina.** Brazil, v. 37, n. 12, p. 667-670. Dec. 2009.

SINGH, N et al. Efficacy of metformin in improving glycaemic control & perinatal outcome in gestational diabetes mellitus: A non-randomized study. **Indian J Med Res.** India.V. 145, n. 5, p. 623-628, May. 2017.

SPAIGHT C et al. Gestational Diabetes Mellitus. **Endocrine Development.** V. 31, p. 163-168.2016.

SOUZA, Gomes de et al. Pregnancy and diabetes: relationship between nutritional status and glycemic control. **Revista Brasileira em Promoçâo da Saù**. v.27, n. 4, p. 1-9. 2014.

SU, DF; WANG, XY. Metformin vs insulin in the management of gestational diabetes: a systematic review and meta-analysis. **Diabetes Res Clin Pract**.v. 104, n.3, p. 353-7, Jun.2014.

SUGIYAMA, T et al. Pregnancy outcomes of gestational diabetes mellitus according to pre-gestational BMI in a retrospective multi-institutional study in Japan. **Endocrine Journal.** Japan, v.61, n. 4,p. 373-80.2016.

TEIXEIRA et al. Nutritional care in gestational diabetes: case report. **Gep News**, Maceió, v.1, n.2, p.32-35, apr./jun. 2017.

Institute of Medicine (IOM). Nutrition during Pregnancy and Lactation: an implementation guide. National Academy Press; Washington (DC), 1992.

WAHABI, H A et al. Pre-pregnancy care for women with pre-gestational diabetes mellitus: a systematic review and meta-analysis. **Nutrition Journal**. n. 12. 2012.

WATSON, W. J. Herceptin (trastuzumab) therapy during preganancy: association with reversible anhydramnios. **Obstetrics & Gynecology,** Danvers, v. 105, n. 3, p. 642-643. 2005.

WEELDEN, Van et al. Long-Term Effects of Oral Antidiabetic Drugs During Pregnancy on Offspring: A Systematic Review and Meta-analysis of Follow-up Studies of RCTs. **Diabetes Ther**. Amsterdam. 2018.

World Health Organization. Definition, diagnosis and classification of diabetes mellitus and its complications: report of a WHO consultation. Geneva: World Health Organization, 1999.

VANLALHRUAII, et al. How safe is metformin when initiated in early pregnancy? A retrospective 5-year study of pregnant women with gestational diabetes mellitus from India. **Diabetes Res Clin Pract.** V. 37, p. 47-55. Mar, 2018.

VOORMOLEN DN et al. Effectiveness of continuous glucose monitoring during diabetic pregnancy (GlucoMOMS trial); a randomized controlled trial. **BMC Pregnancy Childbirth**. Dec. 2012.

YANG ZY. Diet and nutrition interventions prevent gestational diabetes mellitus.

Zhonghua Yu Fang Yi Xue Za Zhi. V. 52, n.1, p. 101-109. China. Jan. 2018.

YAMASHITA, H et al. Factors associated with patients with gestational diabetes in Japan being at increased risk of requiring intensive care. **Int J Gynaecol Obstet.** V. 140, n. 2, p. 170-174. Japan. Feb. 2018.

ZIEGLER A, et al. Long-term protective effect of lactation on the development of type 2 diabetes in women with recent gestational diabetes mellitus. **Diabetes.** v. 61. n. 12, p.3167-71. 2012.

Available at: www.diabetes.org.br/ebook/component/k2/item/37-capitulo-3- resistencia-a-insulina-no-diabetes-gestacional-implicacoes-clinicas ? Accessed Jul 30, 2018.

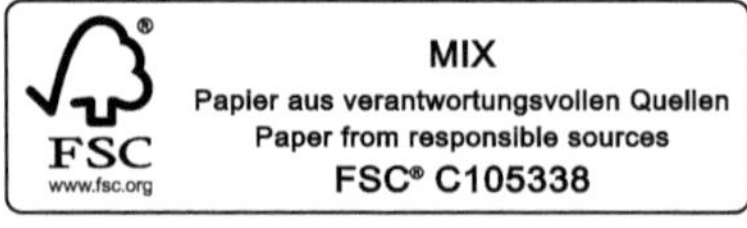